"Cla
and
the
maki

—**Toni Quinn Bankston, LCSW-BACS**, child and family trauma therapist, CEO of Baton Rouge Children's Advocacy Center, and senior faculty and consultant for The Center for Mind-Body Medicine

"Claire Michaels Wheeler brilliantly succeeds in addressing a critical issue—how to cope with stress. This essential framework is a must-read for all those who struggle with the stresses of daily life. Her insights into the biology of stress, particularly the neuroscience, present a blueprint for understanding why stress management is a vital part of our health and happiness."

—**Katherine Grill, PhD**, CEO and cofounder of Neolth, professor at the California Institute of Integral Studies, and behavioral neuroscientist and integrative specialist

"This book is a journey to your inner self, and enhances the understanding of your environment. Science is linked with your body and mind. It teaches you how to understand and analyze your stressors, and to address them in an objective and practical way. Claire Michaels Wheeler's book helped me to recognize my anxiety triggers, and to develop coping mechanisms. To apply the mind-body approach is liberating, and will help you develop more inner strength."

—**Carole Zen Ruffinen, MPH,** pharmacist, and project coordinator for Doctors Without Borders

POCKET THERAPY for STRESS

CLAIRE MICHAELS WHEELER, MD, PHD

New Harbinger Publications, Inc.

PUBLISHER'S NOTE

This publication is designed to provide accurate and authoritative information in regard to the subject matter covered. It is sold with the understanding that the publisher is not engaged in rendering psychological, financial, legal, or other professional services.

Distributed in Canada by Raincoast Books

Copyright © 2020 by Claire Michaels Wheeler
New Harbinger Publications, Inc.
5674 Shattuck Avenue
Oakland, CA 94609
www.newharbinger.com

Cover design by Sara Christian; Acquired by Elizabeth Hollis Hansen; Edited by Marisa Solís; Text design by Michele Waters and Amy Shoup

All Rights Reserved

Printed in the United States of America
Library of Congress Cataloging-in-Publication Data on file

Printed in the United States of America

22   21   20

10   9   8   7   6   5   4   3   2   1   First Printing

CONTENTS

	INTRODUCTION	1
1	ASSESS YOUR STRESS	17
2	USE FLEXIBLE COPING STRATEGIES	31
3	USE YOUR STRENGTHS	55
4	GET INTO THE FLOW	69
5	USE FOOD AS MEDICINE	87
6	GET INTO YOUR BODY	105
7	EXPRESS YOURSELF	113
8	CONNECT WITH OTHERS	135
9	TRAIN YOUR BRAIN	147
10	RISE ABOVE	157
	STRESS TOOL KIT	165

INTRODUCTION

Stress robs us of so much. It's like a thief in the night (literally, it steals our ability to sleep well). It creeps up on us gradually. We often don't realize stress is an issue until we develop high blood pressure or chronic low-back pain or other symptoms.

If you're already grappling with a medical condition, reducing stress can dramatically alter the course of your illness. If you're not, taking steps to manage your stress levels can help you preserve both your physical and your mental health.

The health benefits of managing stress are undeniable. But there's another reason to do it. Clearing your body and mind of unnecessary stress and tension allows you to thrive. It makes room for creativity and spiritual growth. It frees you to pursue valued activities, build happier relationships, and truly appreciate the strength and vibrancy of your body.

This little book offers ten simple but powerful ways to dramatically decrease the negative effects of stress on your life. Some results will be immediate: less muscle tension, clearer thinking, better sleep. Others will be like money in the bank: changes that will help you live a longer, happier, more fulfilling life, such as in your relationships and diet.

In this book you'll find exercises, questionnaires, and writing prompts that will help you discover:

- what stresses you,
- how to effectively respond to stressors, and
- how you can stress much, much less.

In addition, the "Explore" section at the end of each chapter will take you deeper into the chapter topic. Be sure to dedicate a blank journal or notebook (or use your phone's notes app) as a companion to this book. In it you'll document your insights and log your new stress-busting skills.

What Is Stress?

Stress is a process—an interaction between you and your environment. Most researchers and clinicians define stress as *the internal experience that arises when life's challenges and pressures exceed your perceived ability to cope.* Let's look at this definition closely. First, the situation that arises in you is a physical, emotional, psychological, and social phenomenon. In other words, stress is a *holistic response.* Every part of you—body, mind, spirit, and relationships—is affected by the challenges of daily life. The good news is that each part of you can be called upon as a resource for managing these challenges.

Second, stress is determined by how well you think you can cope. Fortunately, coping is a skill that anyone can improve. Coping is the antidote to stress, and the key to better coping is perception. In other words, the meaning of everything that happens to you is entirely up to you. Within the boundaries of normal human existence, stress is not what happens *to* you, it's what you think and feel *about* what happens to you. This means that you can control the amount of stress in your life. How?

- You can change your thoughts about what's going on around you.

- You can change how you react to what's going on around you.

- You can take charge of the fearful, worried, and anxious thoughts that plague your mind, even when you're in a safe, comfortable situation.

- You can choose to avoid situations that create stress for you.

- You can choose to do things that create peace for you.

In this book, we'll explore simple solutions to the problem of stress, based on the power you have right now to change your thoughts, access your inner reserves of strength and vitality, learn new skills, and make new, healthy connections to the world around you.

Acute vs. Chronic Stress

Generally speaking, there are two kinds of stress: *acute* and *chronic*. Acute (temporary) stress is useful; chronic (long-lasting) stress is less useful and can in fact be harmful.

The *acute stress response*—the immediate, automatic response to a stressful event—is one humans share with all other mammals. It's a survival mechanism that causes profound, nearly instantaneous changes in every body system. The general theme is Danger! Run away!

Immediately after you perceive a threat, your brain starts sending messages and releasing hormones that change your state from relaxed to red alert. Heart rate and blood pressure increase, and blood gets shunted away from your skin and digestive organs and into your brain and the large muscles of your body. All of this helps you figure out how to run to safety and gives you the leg power to do so.

In an ideal scenario, once the threat has passed, all systems return to normal and you're able to relax. Your body is designed to do this automatically. But here's where we humans, with our big brains and vast imaginations, come into trouble. If we keep thinking about the past threat—imagining all the terrible things that could have happened, what our friends would think, how much it would have cost, and on and on—we keep the threat alive. If we get stuck in threatened thinking, we get stuck in the *chronic stress response.*

Breaking the cycle of chronic stress starts in the here and now. For some people, it's helpful to follow up with therapy that will help you make sense of the past. But for everyone, learning simple, effective ways to cope with stress right now is the best way to start.

Why Manage Stress?

You know without being told that it's bad for you when you're pushed too hard, either by yourself or by the world you live in. You also know that it's uncomfortable to have that feeling of stress from day to day. But stress isn't just uncomfortable—it's dangerous to your health. Evidence is mounting to support the strong link between chronic stress and a variety of health problems. Upper respiratory infections, coronary artery disease, autoimmune disorders, poor wound healing, depression: all of these problems and many others are made worse by chronic stress.

Consider the physical changes that happen when a threat appears: heart rate, blood pressure, and muscle tension increase, and digestion becomes disrupted. Over time, these conditions cause excessive wear and tear on the organs involved. The heart has to work harder to keep its rate up and push against elevated blood pressure. Muscles get tired, sore, and crampy from chronic tension. Lower-back pain is a hallmark of chronic stress. And if digestion is frequently disrupted by stress, food can't be digested and absorbed properly. This deprives the body of the nutrients it needs to thrive.

Another way that stress causes wear and tear is by interfering with the restorative process of sleep. Sleep is vitally important for mental and physical health. It's a time when all the body's cells can rest, restore, and repair the damage wrought by the stresses and challenges of the day. If you're having problems sleeping, stress is probably a factor in your insomnia. Learning and practicing stress management skills can promote better sleep, and this book will teach you techniques.

The Mind-Body Approach

Mind-body medicine (MBM) provides us with creative and effective ways to manage the nagging ailments related to chronic stress. MBM brings together the fields of biomedicine, health psychology, public health, nursing, and psychotherapy. It is guided by the premise that mind, body, and spirit are integral parts of a system. Information flows to and from these aspects of a person all the time, and they can't be separated. A stressor that affects the mind also affects the body and spirit. Doing something that helps heal your spirit will also heal your body and mind.

Many of the MBM techniques offered in this book work by changing anxious thought patterns and emotional states to calm ones. This simple shift causes big changes in your body. Your heart rate slows, breathing deepens, muscles relax, and blood flow to your digestive organs increases. Your body gets a break from the constant pressure of stress. Over time, as you practice these techniques, it becomes easier and easier to shift from overdrive to neutral. Your thinking becomes clearer, your body feels better, and life seems more manageable.

As you work through the ten simple solutions to stress in this book, be sure to also access the free bonus materials, including additional exercises and resources, at this book's website: www.newharbinger.com/47643.

Before you dive in, use the following exercise to start clarifying where you are now and where you'd like to go.

Ready to Change?

You'll need your notebook, three sheets of plain white paper, and some pencils, crayons, or markers in a variety of colors.

Now, with your materials gathered, sit in a comfortable spot with a firm surface on which you can draw. You're going to create three images. Read these instructions, do the mental imagery, and then draw. Don't stop to think about what you're drawing. Just move the marker over the paper and allow what wants to emerge to come through. Trust yourself.

Image 1: Close your eyes and scan your body for muscle tension. Take a moment to think about that tension melting away. Think about letting go and making yourself soft and receptive. When you feel a shift, settle into it and ask yourself, *How am I doing?* Allow whatever images come to mind to flow past. Don't latch on to any one idea; just let them flow.

Now, pick up whatever marker appeals to you and start to draw. Just create an image that reflects the answer to the question: *How am I doing?* Continue for a minute or two, no longer. This is meant to be a quick, intuitive exercise.

Image 2: Repeat the calming and centering step you did before drawing your first image. This time, ask yourself, *What bothers me?* Again, take a minute or two to create an image that addresses this question.

Image 3: Repeat the calming and centering step. This time, ask yourself, *What makes me happy now?* Take a minute or two to create an image that addresses this question.

Now, look at your first drawing and answer these questions in your journal.

1. What's the overall tone of the image? What word does it bring up for you when you look at it?

2. What are the prominent features of the image? Are there objects, people, colors, or shapes that catch your eye? Write down what they are.

3. Now look for more subtle aspects of the drawing. Is there a little squiggle or some other indeterminate element that means something to you? Write about it.

Next, do the same for the other two pictures, one at a time.

Now, look at the three images as a group and consider these questions: Are there things they have in common? Did you use similar colors? Do some have more energy than others?

How do they seem to fit together? Write about that.

Now, on a fresh page of your notebook, make three columns. Label the first column "Me: Now." Looking at the first image you drew, make a list of five to ten adjectives and short phrases that describe you currently.

Label the second column "Stressors." Let your second image and the writing you did about it be your guide. Some of the items on this list may be obvious, but chances are that some things you hadn't previously considered stressors will appear on your list.

Label the third column "Resources." Start by looking at the third image and your written analysis of it. Now generate a simple list of the good things in your life.

Take a few moments to reflect on the exercise and write whatever comes to you in your journal.

I recommend doing this exercise every couple of months while you're making changes in your life, and then at least once or twice a year afterward. The more loving, well-intentioned attention you give yourself, the more consciously and mindfully you'll live.

Now let's get to work!

1

ASSESS YOUR STRESS

Here's some good news: by simply reading and learning about stress, you may already be countering its effects on your life. People who enter a stress management program show improvement in their stress levels after just the first informational session—before learning any new skills or strategies. So even if you read only this chapter, you're going to benefit. But I hope you'll stick around to learn all ten skills so you can manage your stress most effectively.

Taking stock of the major events in your life is a good starting point for thinking about the stresses you've encountered. Look at the following list and note which events have happened to you in the last year (write "Y" after the event) or month (write "M" after the event).

RELATIONSHIPS	
Death of spouse or significant other (SO)	
Serious injury or illness in spouse or SO	
Serious injury or illness in your child	
Divorce or separation from SO	
Death of a close family member	
Beginning cohabitation with SO	
Marriage	
New pregnancy	
Birth or adoption of a child	
Child leaving home	
Other	

WORK/FINANCES	
Job loss	
Retirement	
Job transfer	
New job	
Starting school	
Graduation	
Significant conflict at work	
Losing a promotion	
Financial setback	
Financial windfall	
Other	

HEALTH	
Newly diagnosed illness	
Serious injury	
Surgery	
New aches or pains	
Other	
OTHER MAJOR EVENTS	
Moving	
Major vacation	
Major purchase	
Dieting	
New exercise program	
Other	

Now count up the number of challenges you've encountered in the past year and in the past month. It's helpful to look at your stressors in each category as well as your total number of stressors. You may find that your life has been very stable in the areas of work and finance, but turbulent in your relationships or other areas. Noticing this will help you appreciate the stability that you do have in your life while coping with the changes that you're experiencing. In general, the higher your number of stressors, the more likely you are to cope in unhealthy, unconstructive ways, at least in the long run.

This exercise can give you some perspective on the number of stressful life events you've experienced, but it tells only part of the story. The biggest limitation to this approach is that stress is subjective. Each item on the list will have a completely different meaning to—and effect on—each person who experiences it.

So, now let's look at your results with a different twist. From the list, choose the event that had the most significant impact on your life. Take some time to reflect on this event and ask yourself the following questions. Write your answers in your journal.

1. How was my health just before this happened?

2. What was my general mood and state of mind before it happened?

3. In the two to four weeks after this event, did I develop a cold or other health problem?

4. In the two to four weeks after this event, did I develop any new aches or pains?

5. Did my sleep habits change during and after this challenge?

6. Did I have anyone to turn to for emotional support when this was happening?

7. Did my use of alcohol, cigarettes, other drugs, TV, or the computer increase during this situation?

8. How long did it take for me to start to feel normal after this happened?

9. Was I able to find anything positive about the experience? Did I learn anything from it that will help me in the future?

Now, let's consider what your answers may mean for you personally.

Questions 3 and 4: Did you answer yes to either question? If so, you may have a close link between life stresses and your immune strength. You may be carrying a load of chronic stress in your body and mind that make you especially vulnerable to the health effects of stress. Working with some of the mind-body techniques in this book can help you get better control over your responses to stressful events and add to your resilience.

Question 5: Insomnia, or difficulty falling asleep or staying asleep (a yes answer to question 5), is an almost universal response to acute stressors and big challenges. Stressful events often lead to (and are made worse by) anxious thinking.

Sometimes stress-related insomnia is more a matter of physical restlessness and arousal than nonstop thinking. During a stressful time, your sympathetic nervous system is activated more than usual. You have more adrenaline flowing in your veins day and night.

There are some extremely effective ways to manage this. One of the best is physical exercise, which you'll learn how to incorporate into your daily routine in chapter 6.

Question 6: If you answered no to this question, you may need to think about developing a social support system. This sounds daunting, but it doesn't have to be. What you can do is take stock of the relationships you already have in your life and think about how you can make them more mutually supportive.

Being able to connect with other people, from the grocery store checker to your spouse, with more patience and humanity will not only protect you from the ravages of stress, but it will also make other people happier.

There are many ways that relationships can add stress to your life, but these usually involve difficulty setting good boundaries, saying no to demands, and asking for what you want (without whining). Strong, healthy relationships improve your resilience. You'll learn strategies for improving your relationships in chapter 8.

Question 7: For many people, alcohol or fatty foods consumed in moderation is an enjoyable part of life. During stressful periods, however, people tend to use these more, looking for a quick jolt of pleasure that will take them away from the challenges of the present moment. However, it's not just pleasure that you may be seeking. You might be using substances to try to counteract the symptoms of stress—for example, using caffeine during the day to stay awake and productive when you're not getting enough sleep, or using sleeping pills when you're having difficulty falling asleep. Throughout this book you'll learn healthy coping strategies, and chapter 5 offers tips to reduce stress with healthier eating.

Questions 8 and 9: These questions address your resiliency. How long does it take you to recover from a stressful incident? Can you survive a stressful event and feel that, even though you didn't ask for it and wouldn't choose to experience it again, you still got something positive out of it? When you're in the thick of a crisis, finding or creating some kind of positive meaning gives you strength to see things through. Chapter 10 discusses the strength that can be derived from a spiritual practice, while chapters 3 and 4 offer strategies for gaining strength from things you do well or enjoy doing.

Explore

To get a better sense of how stress is affecting you now, visit www.newharbinger.com/47643 and download the worksheet titled Evaluate Your Stress Symptoms. You will rate your current stress level, and your score will help you understand how serious your situation is.

Next, take out your journal and reflect on what you learned about your stress challenges and responses. What insights about your stress did you gain from this chapter? Consider its impact on your health, mood, sleep, social support, substance use, and personal resiliency.

2

USE FLEXIBLE COPING STRATEGIES

Coping and stress go hand in hand. Coping is anything you do to relieve any unsettling effects of stressful events. Many of the things we think of as bad habits are actually misguided coping strategies, those that lead to more problems and more stress. These unhelpful coping responses include watching too much television, drinking alcohol, procrastinating, and eating comfort foods.

Let's start with this abbreviated version of the COPE questionnaire, developed by Charles Carver with Michael Scheier and Jagdish Weintraub.

Rate how often you use each of the following possible ways of dealing with stressful events in your life. Use the following scale:

I don't do this at all	1
I do this a little bit	2
I do this in moderation	3
I do this a lot	4

1. I turn to work and other activities to take my mind off things.
2. I concentrate my efforts on doing something about the situation that's bothering me.
3. I say to myself, "This isn't real."
4. I use alcohol or drugs to make myself feel better.
5. I get emotional support from others.

6. I take action to try to make the situation better.

7. I refuse to believe that the situation has happened.

8. I say things to let my unpleasant feelings escape.

9. I get help and advice from other people.

10. I use alcohol or other drugs to help me get through it.

11. I try to see the situation in a different light, to make it seem more positive.

12. I try to come up with a strategy about what to do.

13. I get comfort and understanding from someone.

Use Flexible Coping Strategies

14. I look for something good in what's happening.
15. I do something to think about it less, like going to the movies, watching TV, reading, daydreaming, sleeping, or shopping.
16. I accept the reality of the fact that it has happened.
17. I express my negative feelings.
18. I try to find comfort in my religious or spiritual beliefs.
19. I try to get advice or help from other people about what to do.
20. I try to learn to live with it.
21. I think hard about what steps to take.
22. I pray or meditate.

Now, consider what types of coping strategies you rely on:

STRESS RESPONSES	COPING STRATEGY
1 and 15	Self-distraction
2 and 6	Active coping
3 and 7	Denial
4 and 10	Substance use
5 and 13	Use of emotional social support
9 and 19	Use of instrumental social support
8 and 17	Venting
11 and 14	Positive reframing
12 and 21	Planning
16 and 20	Acceptance
18 and 22	Transcendence

As you read the rest of this chapter, consider which of your go-to coping strategies you'd like to replace with healthier ones.

Coping is a two-stage process of appraisal—that is, *making judgments about what's happening and what you're going to do about it*. The first step is *primary appraisal*, in which you decide whether something is a threat to you or your interests. The *secondary appraisal* concerns whether there's anything you can do to change the situation to minimize bad outcomes and increase the possibility of positive outcomes.

In the primary appraisal, you determine what's at stake in the situation. In a traffic jam, what's at stake may be being late to work. As the stressors become more serious, as in the case of a medical diagnosis, the stakes get higher and the potential for distress increases. Primary appraisals can run the gamut from total denial of the significance of the event to overt catastrophizing. Primary appraisals are important because they set the stage for your responses.

Track Your Primary Appraisals

For this exercise, you'll need to carry your journal with you for an entire day. Ideally, this would be a typical day in which you take care of your usual responsibilities. Begin the day by setting the intention to be aware of everything that bothers you for the entire day and to write it down in your notebook. You can download an example of a complete day at www.newharbinger.com/47643.

Continue listing stressors as they arise throughout the day. Remember, these can be things that are actually happening or simply thoughts that cause you to feel uncomfortable, worried, or anxious.

Now, find some time as soon as possible after your observation day to sit down with your list. For each item on the list, answer two questions in your notebook:

1. What is at stake here? What can I lose or how can this harm me?

2. How likely is it that something bad will happen as a result of this event?

Chances are, for many of the potential stressors you encounter each day, the actual threat to your well-being is not as great as it may have felt at the time. With practice, you will learn to ask these two questions in the moment, as the stress is occurring. This way, you can stop automatic stress responses before they happen.

Working with primary appraisals involves putting the events of daily life into a larger perspective. It's also helpful to explore the roots of your negative valuations of life's events. There are many reasons that relatively minor, harmless events can trigger a sense of threat. Some possibilities include:

- Minor events may remind you of bigger stressors and traumas from the past.

- Daily stressors can trigger memories of painful childhood incidents.

- Daily challenges can tap into erroneous beliefs about a vulnerability from the past.

- Stressful events can sometimes be seen as part of a bigger pattern of loss, helplessness, or persecution that doesn't exist.

Going through your list again, ask yourself whether any of these—or any other unhelpful assumptions—are affecting how you look at things. If you find that you tend to overestimate the possible negative impact of relatively minor life events, it can be helpful to create a verbal cue that you can say to yourself whenever these things come up. Some examples are:

How interesting!

At least it's not _____. This is manageable.

No big deal.

Humor can be very helpful here. This is not to say that you should minimize the importance of life's stressors to the point that you don't take care of yourself and deal with problems as they arise. The point is to recognize that most of these things, even if they happen repeatedly, are transient and really don't matter much in the big scheme of things.

Another valuable resource when making primary appraisals is the people in your life who are supportive. Talking about what's bothering you can help you reassess the level of threat in the situation, for better or worse. It can provide a reality check of whether your perceptions of threat are realistic, given the perspective of someone you trust.

Track Your Secondary Appraisals

The secondary appraisal involves answering two questions about an event that, in your primary appraisal, you have decided is a threat to you. Select one or more events, then write down your responses to the following questions:

1. Do I have any control over this situation, and can I change it to make it less threatening?

2. Can I handle the emotions I feel in response to this event and its consequences?

The secondary appraisal can be something that happens in your conscious mind, or it can be an automatic response to your primary appraisal. If you take control over making the secondary appraisal, however, you can be in charge of the coping strategies you use.

It's important to be able to tell the difference between situations you can control and those you can't, because a false feeling of control can lead to great emotional distress and interfere with acceptance, something that helps you thrive in the face of stress. This is another way that social support is beneficial. Friends and family can help you figure out whether you have control and what resources you have available to you for coping.

Most people have developed coping strategies that they've used for years, and they tend to use them in response to all the stresses they're exposed to. For example, some people tend to become confrontational whenever they feel anxious, scared, or angry. This approach may be helpful in some situations, like dealing with shady salespeople, but counterproductive when you're stopped for a speeding ticket.

Other people have a more passive coping style. They rarely seem angry and tend to ignore problems, hoping they'll pass. This can be helpful for stressors that are temporary and minor, like travel delays, but can be a real problem if the stressor is serious and requires action, like filing taxes.

The most beneficial approach is to be as flexible as possible with your coping strategies—and to learn when to apply which skill from your repertoire.

Secondary appraisals—deciding whether you can exert any control to improve a situation and evaluating whether you can cope with it—involve a *thinking component* and a *feeling component.* This is also true of coping strategies. Some responses to stressful events are primarily cognitive; others are more emotional. Over and over again, all day, you are using some combination of cognitive and emotional strategies, often without even knowing you're doing it. Imagine how much more effective you can be if you cultivate a variety of coping skills and learn when, where, and how to use them.

Problem Solving

Problem-solving coping skills are most appropriate in situations over which you have at least some control. Problem solving is a logical response when your secondary appraisal tells you, *Yes, there's something you can do about what's happening to make it less of a threat.* The following are some examples of problem solving:

"Planful" problem solving: Making a plan to confront a problem helps you define the problem in concrete terms and tends to bring the possible negative outcomes down to earth. Try taking pen to paper and writing down a series of steps you can take to address the problem. Allow yourself to be unrealistic, fanciful, and even playful in the steps you could take.

Confrontive coping: You can think of this as sticking up for yourself. Taken to an extreme, this type of coping can alienate people and pose a risk to your social support network. The key is to direct your confrontational energy where it will be most helpful. For example, if you're upset with your boss, communicate your concerns directly rather than taking your frustration out on your coworkers.

Information seeking: This is an active coping technique that can alleviate stress by reducing uncertainty. It's generally considered a helpful approach, especially when the stressor is a health problem, but there are some caveats. First, information seeking may work best for challenges that are short term and for which information is readily available. For longer-term stressors, an emphasis on information seeking can lead to a type of hypervigilance that can become stressful in itself.

Mental stimulation: Mental simulation is seeing, feeling, and imagining yourself successfully managing a stressful situation. In a relaxed state, you can take yourself through the event (for example, a major exam or a scary confrontation with someone) and see yourself staying calm, making good choices, and avoiding harm.

Instrumental social support: Instrumental social support is practical help when you need it. Perhaps you need a ride to the hospital or a short-term loan. Having one or more people in your life on whom you can count for these things is a real benefit.

Emotion Regulation

When a situation is a threat that is mostly, if not completely, out of your control, sometimes your only recourse is to manage your emotional responses and ride it out. It's very important to be able to minimize your level of emotional distress in the face of stress without denying or suppressing your thoughts and feelings.

Emotional social support: Emotional social support comes in the form of someone in your life who you trust, who you can talk to about your problems. This gives you a feeling of connectedness that helps avert loneliness. Also, emotional social support helps you create a logical story about the problem and make a realistic assessment of the resources available to you for coping.

Accessing and venting emotions: Emotions can take on a life of their own. The key to emotional venting is to allow a free flow of what you're feeling but to avoid getting preoccupied with the emotional consequences of the problem at the expense of working on solving the problem. Physical exercise is an extremely good method of discharging emotional energy.

Meaning-Making

Meaning-based coping is a set of skills recently recognized as effective coping tools. It's a way to seek personal growth and wisdom through life's difficult times.

Positive reinterpretation and growth: Finding the silver lining in a dark cloud can be a blessing. It's possible to look at stress and problems as learning experiences, even when you endure a great loss. This becomes easier when you cultivate an attitude of acceptance of things you can't control.

Religion or spirituality: The physical and mental health benefits of religiousness and spirituality have been documented extensively in recent medical literature. Part of these benefits seems to come from the way a transcendent perspective on life helps people cope with problems. Putting everyday issues into a larger perspective helps them seem smaller and more manageable.

Making comparisons: No matter how bad things get, it's always possible to imagine that someone else is worse off than you are, or that things could get worse. If your house burns down, at least nobody was hurt. If you lose a breast to cancer, at least you're still alive. If you lose your job, at least you have your health. Thoughts like these can help you stay engaged in active coping because you're thinking about the problem without being defeated by it.

Finding side benefits: You can learn from the bad things that happen to you. You can become more appreciative of the good things in your life. You can learn to embrace every day that you're given. All of these side benefits and more are the hidden gifts of stress and trauma, and it's up to you to find and appreciate them.

Explore

What insights about your coping style and strategies did you gain from this chapter? Take out your journal and respond to the following prompts:

- My main coping style is…

- A time when my coping style or strategy was really effective…

- A time when my coping style or strategy was really not effective…

- Coping strategies I tend to overuse are…

- Coping strategies I could stand to use more often are…

Remember: most coping styles and strategies are neither inherently "good" nor "bad"—they're just more or less helpful, healthy, or effective.

3

USE YOUR STRENGTHS

Being happy and being debilitated by stress are often seen as incompatible states of being. There is no way to avoid stress and challenge in life, but it is entirely possible to maintain a sense of happiness and well-being even in the most difficult circumstances.

Positive psychology is dedicated to figuring out what people do well and how to build on their strengths so that individuals and societies can become happier and more constructive. Let's focus on the virtues and strengths that are most useful in coping with stress.

Optimism

Optimism is a stance toward life that continually allows for good outcomes. In recent years, it has been linked to better health, better performance at work and school, longer life, and more happiness. Optimism seems to exert its benefits in several ways. One is through its effects on mood. People who can endure stress and still maintain a positive emotional tone reap many rewards. Good mood seems to go along with better flexibility in thinking about your options, and it promotes generosity and social responsibility. There are many health benefits to social support, and optimism, with its attendant positive mood states, may encourage people to create and sustain more supportive relationships with others. Optimism also inspires people to engage in more self-care.

Optimists can be defined by the way they explain the things that happen to them. When something bad happens, an optimist tends to explain it in terms of causes that are external (not internal) to the self, transient (not stable), and specific to the situation (not global). A pessimistic person would make the opposite attributions.

Here's an example of optimism at work: I'm driving to work on a rainy day. I'm running a little late, so I'm hurrying but not speeding. On a bend in the road, I skid out and end up with my car in the ditch. An optimist would explain the situation this way: *The road is slippery* (low internality) *because it's raining today* (low stability). *The bend in the road is particularly sharp and hard to navigate when the road is slippery* (low globality). Now let's look at how a pessimist would explain the same situation: *I was driving too fast because I didn't manage my time well today* (high internality). *I am always running late* (high stability), *and this is only one of the stupid things that have happened because I'm so bad at managing my time* (high globality).

Can you learn to be more optimistic? Research suggests that you can. When something bad happens, pay attention to your thoughts. Do you assume that the situation happened because of something about you or something you did? Is it something that *always* happens to you? Is it just one example of the kind of thing that happens to you? Ask yourself whether there's another possible explanation that's external, transient, and specific to the situation.

Self-Efficacy

Self-efficacy is the belief that, even in the most difficult circumstances, you can take care of yourself. It's the conviction that you have some control over the events of your life. This quality goes hand in hand with optimism. Where optimism helps you develop your expectations for the future, building self-efficacy can improve your confidence that you are capable of meeting those expectations, even when things are hard to handle. Self-efficacy is situation specific—that is, you can have high self-efficacy about your capabilities as a student but low self-efficacy in the area of romantic relationships.

Having high self-efficacy motivates you to work harder and be more persistent in reaching your goals. The good news is that you can learn to have more self-efficacy in any area of your life. How do you do this? There are several well-documented ways. The first step is to be very specific about what you want to feel more confident about. This is often easiest if you think of it in terms of a goal. Let's say you want to start exercising regularly. How can you build your self-efficacy with respect to that goal, and thereby increase your chances of accomplishing it? Here's how:

Provide yourself with the experience of success. Set small goals that gradually build to your ultimate desired outcome.

Live vicariously. Find examples of people who have accomplished similar goals.

Let yourself be persuaded. You think you need to get more exercise to be healthier? Why not ask your doctor what she thinks? I can almost guarantee you that she will help you by telling you it's a great idea.

Pay attention to how you feel. Something inside you is motivating you to take up walking. What is it? Do you feel anxious about your health and the possible consequences of being out of shape? Pay attention to that anxiety and see how much better you feel after you take that walk.

Choosing Happiness

Happiness can be seen as a choice you make in life. For many people, it's the only thing really worth striving for. Focusing on your strengths is one way to cultivate true happiness. Looking at the research on happiness, Jason Satterfield, from the University of California, San Francisco, made the following observations:

- Happiness seems to occur most often in people who have good social support, are married, have religion or spirituality in their lives, and tend to be more extroverted than introverted.

- Unhappiness seems to occur more often in people who value money, status, prestige, and occupational success than in people who value relationships above all other things.

- Things that seem to have little or no effect on a person's happiness include age, gender, income (above the level at which the most basic needs are met), and physical attractiveness.

Here's an interesting exercise to try. First, make a list of the things you think are most important in life, in your heart and mind and ideals. Number these priorities and arrange them in a list, with the most important at the top. Next, think about your average week. Make a list of broad categories of what you do during the week: working, watching television, being with your family, going to church, and so on. Now, arrange this list with the activity that takes the most time at the top and the one that takes the least time at the bottom. Compare your two lists. Are you spending enough time on the things you value most? It's especially valuable to consider how you use your time outside of work.

Think about whether what you do in your free time aligns with what you truly care about.

You can further explore the idea of virtues and strengths by visiting the positive psychology website https://www.viastrengths.org.

Building Happiness

First, in your notebook write about how you've been feeling for the past couple of weeks. After you've written for a few minutes, stop and answer these questions in your notebook.

1. Overall, how happy have you been?

2. Overall, how well have you been getting along with the people close to you?

3. How have you been sleeping?

4. How well have you been taking care of your health needs?

5. What are your expectations for your life in the next month or so?

6. What are your expectations for your life in the next year or two?

7. How would you rate your overall quality of life?

During the next week, do one of the following activities:

Gratitude visit: Write a letter of gratitude to a person who has been especially kind to you and who you feel you haven't properly thanked. After you've written the letter, deliver it in person.

Three good things in life: Every night, sit down with your journal and write down three things that went well that day. In addition, write down the causes of each of the good things. Then write a brief explanation of each cause.

You at your best: In your notebook, write a story about a time in your life when you were at your absolute best. Make it about a page long, and go into detail about why you were at your best.

Use your strengths: Go to https://www.authentichappiness.org and take the VIA survey of character strengths. When you get the results, make a list of your top five strengths in your notebook. During the next week, see if you can consciously use these strengths as often as possible in daily life.

At the end of the week, go back to the seven questions. What changes do you see?

Explore

For each of the top five strengths you identified in this chapter:

- Write about a time *in the past week* when you consciously chose to use that strength.

- Write about a time *in your life so far* when that strength helped get you through a rough patch.

4

GET INTO THE FLOW

Sometimes it seems that life comes at you in a rush. The older you get, the more pronounced the sense of life flashing by becomes. In itself, this change in your sense of time can become stressful in practical ways, but it's also stressful in the existential sense. It can create a kind of despair to feel your life slipping away without your being able to enjoy, savor, and deeply experience it.

Surely there must be a way, in the midst of all you have to do, to slow down and be in the flow of life as it's happening. The good news is that, yes, there are ways you can rein in the rush of time and be fully present in daily life. How? The two most powerful ways I know of to do that are by seeking flow and cultivating mindfulness.

Flow

Flow is the state of being in which creativity occurs. Flow can happen during many different activities. Have you ever been so involved in doing something that you lost track of time? Maybe you've had an experience when one moment flowed into the next, and you were thinking only about what you were doing? Take a moment and ask yourself what things you have done that engaged your full attention in a pleasurable, rhythmic way, without being stressful. That is flow.

The flow state has several characteristics that refer to both the task itself and the mind state of the person performing the task. Let's consider each of these characteristics.

Clear goals: In flow, you always know what needs to be done. For example, the musician knows what notes to play next. In flow, goals create structure for your experiences, but actually accomplishing them is not the reason for engaging in the activity. It's a lovely paradox, really, balancing the act of setting goals for structure without being strongly attached to the outcome of the activity. This is what happens when the reason for doing something is the doing, not the end result.

Immediate feedback: In order to stay engaged in a process, whether it's at work or at play, you need to know how you're doing. In some arenas, like academia, this information is easy to come by. In other endeavors, the feedback comes from within. Setting goals creates an opportunity to give yourself feedback. In flow states, there is always some form of immediate feedback.

Balance between challenge and skills: In order for an activity to trigger the flow state, it has to offer an optimal balance of challenge and skill. When you're flowing, you're neither frustrated nor bored. You're riding the edge of your abilities, completing a somewhat difficult task you have the talent to finish. Goal setting and feedback are part of this as well. Something as simple as emptying the dishwasher can be flow-enhancing if you set the goal to get it done as smoothly and efficiently as possible.

Merging of action and awareness: In flow, action and awareness are merged. You are in the moment, fully mindful of what you are doing. We're going to focus on mindfulness later in this chapter, but for now, consider that you can pay attention to what's happening to your body, mind, and spirit during any activity.

No distractions: In the flow state, distractions are excluded from consciousness, because a person in flow is engaged in intense concentration on the present. When you embrace the present moment this way, you are relieved of nagging fears, performance anxiety, and worries about the past or future.

No self-consciousness: In flow, debilitating self-consciousness disappears. The constant self-criticism, which can be very stressful, stops. Paradoxically, you become more competent, more relaxed, and therefore more attractive and easy to be with.

Distorted sense of time: During flow, your sense of time becomes distorted. You can be lost in a moment that seems to last forever, or you can look up from a project and realize that hours have passed.

Autotelic experience: Living life in flow means transforming more and more of your daily tasks from things you have to do to things you want to do. The doing—not the result—becomes the thing. That is *autotelic experience*. "Autotelic," which comes from Greek, means that something is an end in itself. Some activities—such as art, music, and sports—are usually autotelic; there is little reason for doing them except to feel the experience they provide. In many ways, the secret to a happy life is to learn to get flow from as many mundane or obligatory things as possible.

Finding Flow Every Day

Flow isn't something you are taught; it's a state that your body and mind want to be in. Begin with one task you do each day. To make it easy, choose something you do in your free time for fun, such as going for a walk, playing a musical instrument, or doing a hobby. Chances are, you already experience some degree of flow while doing what you enjoy. Next time you do this activity, pay attention to each of the dimensions of flow: goals, feedback, and present-moment absorption. Notice what it is about the activity that pleases you. Allow yourself to become immersed in the activity with no distractions.

Next, seek flow with another task, one that doesn't usually bring you a lot of joy, like paying your bills or washing the kitchen floor. Again, see if you can apply some of the principles of flow to this activity.

Keep trying to find flow, and it will begin to come naturally, because you are hardwired for it. It's simply a matter of getting your busy mind out of the way so you can experience life directly.

Mindfulness

Mindfulness is an aspect of flow, but it stands on its own as a way of experiencing life in the present moment. In simplest terms, mindfulness is the act of paying attention to your life as it unfolds, without placing value judgments on anything that happens.

It's a natural human tendency to judge and evaluate everything around us. It's a basic survival instinct that often serves us well. Being mindful is not walking around in a perpetual state of bliss, examining each flower as if the secrets of the universe lay within it. Mindfulness is a here-and-now, hands-on approach to living that makes daily life richer and more instructive. If you approach life as a learning experience, an opportunity to grow and move toward wisdom and grace, you will almost certainly become a more mindful person. Mindfulness is a skill that can help you slow down, cue in, and be an active participant in every moment of your life.

In their review of the research on the effects of meditation on the brain, Rael Cahn and John Polich speculate that one of the reasons meditation helps reduce the symptoms of depression and stress is that it encourages the individual to see negative thoughts as something separate from the self. Simply saying to yourself, *This is only a thought I'm having right now and it will pass*, acknowledges the temporary nature of all thoughts.

Emotional stability goes hand in hand with detaching from the content of your thoughts. Simply giving yourself time between observing a thought and reacting to it can prevent many emotional dips in the course of a single day. The first step is to realize that thoughts are simply content—words and little stories. You can pay attention to them, perhaps even heed them and act on them, but you need not allow them to determine your emotional state. That is something you can practice and get very good at.

Quieting Your Mind

A quiet mind is a blessing you can grant yourself with practice. Can you remember a time when all you were doing was sitting, and maybe looking? Hearing sounds, tensing your body, feeling your breath but not creating a narrative about what was happening? Can you remember times when you were simply being, not doing anything, not even meditating or "relaxing"? When you are still but highly observant, not bothered by assessments (good or bad, okay or not okay) but simply allowing everything around you to be what it is, you are in a meditative state.

An Anytime Mindfulness Practice

Here is a good way to begin practicing mindfulness. Find a time when you can take ten minutes to yourself. You do not have to be in a darkened room; you can be outside, in the lobby of a large office building or a hotel, on your front porch, even in your car (if it's not moving). All you need is to sit and be fairly confident that you won't be interrupted for a few minutes.

Now, get comfortable in your seat. Uncross your legs, if you're able to. With both feet on the ground and your hands in your lap, check your whole body once more to make sure you can relax.

Now, start thinking about the fact that you're breathing. Just notice. You might think, *Hey, guess what? There's air flowing in and out of me every few seconds. And the air is a bit cool as it flows into my nose and into my throat. I can feel my chest expanding as the air fills it.* Just notice this for a minute or so. If your mind wanders away from the miracle that is your breath, just let go of whatever your mind has got its teeth into and return your attention to the air flowing in and out, in and out.

Now, start to pay attention to what is going on around you. This is a shift you need to make carefully, because you might find your mind flooded with words about what things look like and whether things are okay. If this happens, gently return your attention to your breath. Say to yourself, *Air in, air out*, with the movement of your breath until you can be curiously attentive to the world around you without the running commentary.

Simple awareness is something humans are born with—babies and toddlers use it all the time. They're just observing. As you practice this, you'll slowly develop the ability to shift into simple awareness a few times each day. It's a very different way of being in the world, one that short-circuits stress.

Eventually, you'll want to make the connection between occasionally practicing simple awareness in the world and practicing it continually with respect to your own thoughts and perceptions. Think about this: you can observe your thoughts and actions the way you observe the world, without constant judgment, and simply allow yourself to be as you are.

Meditation for Maniacs

Are you a person who always has something to do? Chances are, this describes you (or you wouldn't be reading a book about stress management!). Life is demanding, pulling you in all different directions. You, like most people, probably feel like a maniac at least some of the time. It's vital to your physical, emotional, and psychological health to break the spiral of intensity. You can learn to stop the madness for a few minutes and then dive right back in, refreshed and better able to cope.

One excellent way to do this is to use the *three-breath technique*. You can do this anytime, anywhere. All you have to do is recognize the signs of stress. As soon as you start to feel overwhelmed, stop for a minute. Say to yourself, *I need a break*. Take three breaths with your full attention on each one. Start by fully exhaling. Then calmly, carefully observe the next breath coming in. Feel it expanding inside you, and think to yourself, *Thank you*. Hold the breath for an instant, and then let it out slowly, thinking to yourself, *Let go*. Repeat this twice more. Don't cheat yourself. You have time to do this carefully, slowly, and mindfully.

Mindful Walking

I can't write about meditation, mindfulness, and flow without mentioning my favorite type of meditation: mindful walking. This is simply the act of taking a very slow walk during which you pay close attention to everything that happens. Start by coordinating your breath with your steps. Take a step as you inhale, take a step as you exhale. Continue this for a while, noticing how each foot touches the ground, how your chest expands, whether or not it feels awkward to be walking so slowly.

Gradually, turn your attention to your surroundings. It's amazing to discover how many details you've been missing. If you like mindful walking, you might enjoy tai chi, qigong, or yoga.

Explore

Using the information from this chapter, reflect:

- Which of the methods in this chapter did you try: finding flow, simple awareness, the three-breath technique, or mindful walking? What was it like to try them?

- If you used a method that seemed to work, make a plan to practice it for at least a month. Setting a reminder on your phone can help you make it part of your life, so the skill is there when you need it.

- If you like the idea of one of these methods, but it didn't seem to work right away when you tried it, still practice it for a month. It might grow on you. And you will be developing the skill in the process.

5

USE FOOD AS MEDICINE

There are profound and intimate connections between diet and stress. The relationship runs both ways: less-than-optimal nutrition can make you more susceptible to stress, and stress can affect your ability to choose healthy food, digest it, and absorb nutrients.

Food is something most people take for granted. Food is essential to life, but it's also fraught with emotional and social baggage. Because our culture values physical appearance, many people spend their lives trying to meet an aesthetic ideal that isn't realistic for the average person. At the same time, we're presented with more and more access to fatty, high-sodium, nutrient-poor food. The mixed messages from advertising and entertainment can create a lot of stress.

The time pressures of jobs, childcare, home management, and all the other requirements of everyday life make it very appealing to simply pull a box out of the freezer, pop it in the microwave, and call it dinner. In the short run, this may seem like a good way to save time and reduce stress. However, when you sacrifice the daily rituals of buying, preparing, and slowly and consciously eating food, you miss out on the potential social, emotional, and physical advantages of eating while relaxed.

Portion sizes at fast-food restaurants are two to five times bigger now than they were thirty years ago. In the past decade, the average portion size for meals eaten at home has also dramatically increased. This amounts to a tremendous increase in the average daily intake of calories and is surely a major contributor to the obesity epidemic.

Additionally, the news media frequently present reasons to be afraid of food, from mad cow disease to salmonella contamination to pesticide residues on produce. Often, the reports are unfounded, rely on inadequate research, or exaggerate a minor risk. Yet people respond with fear and confusion, experiencing even more of the stress already inherent in modern life. It's important to keep food scares in perspective. For the most part, our food supply is safe. The best protection is to eat a wide variety of foods in their most natural form.

Stress Affects Your Diet

Stress can have a powerful effect on appetite and food cravings. When you're stressed, your nutritional needs change. Yet this is when most people shift into emergency eating mode. Rushing, eating fast food, eating processed foods, eating standing up or in front of the television: all these habits only make stress more harmful to the body and mind.

Some stress-related overeating is simply a habitually pleasant activity. Consider the psychological and emotional reasons you might turn to food when you're feeling overwhelmed. In our society, food is readily available, it's very tasty, and it's cheap. It provides an experience of immediate gratification. Eating is a social endeavor, a pleasure we can share with family, friends, and coworkers. Sharing food and drinking high-calorie beverages like beer are pleasant activities that provide relief from the daily grind. But consider the following:

Stress makes you eat more. In the recovery phase of chronic stress, cortisol works to protect the body during a long-term challenge by increasing fat storage. It does this by stimulating a desire for pleasurable activity—including eating. This makes sense when you think about human beings living anywhere but in an affluent, developed country. Under conditions of chronic stress, these people would want to keep their strength up by eating more. In twenty-first-century America, chronic stress tends to trigger appetite, and food is everywhere. This appears to be a major contributor to rising levels of overweight and obesity. But this is only part of the story.

Stress makes you crave sugar and fat. Chronic stress seems to affect not only how much you eat but also what you choose to eat. Cortisol and the emotional effects of stress tend to increase the desire for foods that are sweet and high in fat. Sweet, fatty foods can induce a release of the brain's natural opiates, molecules that decrease pain and create euphoria. This momentary rise in brain opioids can actually create addiction, and withdrawal can occur if the supply of sugar is cut off.

Stress directs fat storage to the abdomen. High levels of cortisol cause more fat to be stored in the fat cells of the abdomen. Called visceral fat, it poses a very real danger to cardiovascular health because of its effects on blood sugar and blood cholesterol. People with large amounts of visceral fat are at higher risk of heart disease, type 2 diabetes, high blood pressure, and premature death. Abdominal fat often comes from foods high in carbohydrates and fat, like pastries and ice cream, which tend to be used as comfort food. Eating more high-carbohydrate, high-fat foods makes it more likely that your belly will work to calm your frazzled brain. In this way, you're biochemically rewarded for eating comfort foods and maintaining visceral fat. Indeed, for some people, overeating is an unconscious but real attempt to increase abdominal fat stores because these cells interact with the brain to suppress stress responses and improve mood. The cost of this mood elevation is very high, however, and there are other ways to accomplish this, including taking a thirty-minute walk.

Poor Diet Contributes to Stress

Clearly, stress influences which foods you choose, what your body does with those foods, and how that affects your health. But the equation works the other way too: your diet can affect your stress levels.

Whether you eat too much or are dieting to lose weight, your intake of vital nutrients probably isn't adequate for long-term health. This has everything to do with processed food, food that has been altered to be more palatable (sweeter or saltier), to be quicker or easier to prepare, or to last longer on the shelf. Processing many types of food, especially whole grains, strips it of its nutrients. Most people's diets are deficient in several nutrients—including zinc, vitamin D, and magnesium—that are important for countering the effects of stress. We have the makings of a vicious cycle here, whereby inadequate nutrition is both a trigger and a consequence of stress, leading to higher rates of overweight, obesity, and chronic disease.

When people are on a weight-loss diet or other restricted eating regimen, they're much more likely to overeat in response to stress and distressing emotions. People who are dieting have smaller amounts of natural opioids, the molecules of pleasure in the brain. The brain compensates by becoming more receptive to even small amounts of natural (or synthetic) opioids. A single cookie or other treat causes a release of these substances in the brain, creating a huge craving that may only be satisfied by a binge.

Finally, eating, in and of itself, tends to stimulate the release of cortisol. After a large meal, the stomach is distended by food. The body responds to this by increasing blood pressure and heart rate, classic signs of a stress response. This is a normal response, but it can become problematic when you eat frequently and beyond the point of being satisfied. One way to counteract these effects is to eat more slowly and deliberately, and to focus on the bodily sensations of chewing, swallowing, and sensing the food in your stomach.

Food can be one of your best stress management tools, if you use it wisely. It's okay to eat for comfort, as long as you're choosing foods that create calm nourishment for your body. The comfort level goes up even more if you take the time to prepare the food yourself and serve it simply and beautifully. Eating healthful food slowly and mindfully, in the presence of people you care about, is one of life's great pleasures. Yes, it takes a little more time to eat this way, but the rewards are priceless.

What Should You Eat?

The first thing to consider is the balance of macronutrients you consume each day. Is your diet loaded with simple carbohydrates, manufactured fats, or processed meats? These foods tend to increase the effects of stress on the body. Start by balancing the amounts of protein, carbohydrate, and fat in your diet.

Protein: Protein should come in the form of lean meats and fish, with an emphasis on fish because it also provides the best kind of fats for fighting stress. Other good sources of protein include nonfat or low-fat cottage cheese and yogurt, whey protein, eggs, lentils, and kidney beans.

Fats: You also need a steady flow of good fats (such as fish oil), because they're used by the brain to transform amino acids into neurotransmitters. Avoid trans fats and other factory-made fats in favor of simple, pure olive oil and canola oil.

Carbohydrates: The body absorbs the most tryptophan from a meal or snack that is high in carbohydrates and low in protein. This results in an increase in serotonin levels in the brain, which may lead you to crave this type of food as a form of self-medication when you are anxious or feeling negative emotions. This is okay as long as these cravings are relieved by favoring complex carbohydrates (those found in whole-grain foods, fruits, and vegetables) over simple carbohydrates (the sugars found in juice, candy, and pastries).

Vitamins and minerals: Another important nutrient you need to care for your brain is vitamin C, which is also used to make neurotransmitters. Other nutrients that tend to be depleted when you're under chronic stress are the B vitamins and magnesium.

Vegetables: Vegetables are probably the most neglected and most beneficial foods available to us. One of the best things you can do for yourself is to fall in love with three or four different vegetables and eat them regularly. Simply by eating more vegetables, you can help your body counteract the effects of stress. The U.S. Department of Health and Human Services and the U.S. Department of Agriculture jointly recommend that everyone eat at least two and a half cups of vegetables every day. Most people don't come close to this level.

How Should You Eat?

Mindful eating is the act of slowing down and paying attention while eating. This is an excellent practice for breaking some of the connections between eating and stress. Many problems with overeating come from a sense of needing to hurry up and get to the next thing. It's helpful to reconsider eating and make at least one meal every day an opportunity to slow down and take care of yourself.

A Mindful Snack

Start with a visit to your local grocery store and choose a vegetable or two that you would like to take home and cook and eat. Be picky; choose only pieces that look fresh, smell good, and have good color and texture.

At home, set the intention that you're going to fully appreciate the food you've chosen. Start by washing it and removing any unwanted leaves, stems, or other parts. Notice the color, texture, and smell of the vegetable. Imagine the seeds that were planted, the soil the plant grew in, the sunshine and rain that nurtured it. Try to visualize all the people involved in cultivating and harvesting this food that is now in your kitchen. Consider giving thanks for the miraculous series of events that enable you to be easily and readily fed every day.

Cook the vegetable carefully, being sure not to overcook it. It's done perfectly when the color has peaked in intensity and the texture has become soft enough to chew but not mushy. Choose a nice plate or bowl, and pay attention as you serve. Are you going to put butter on it? Salt? Perhaps it's worthy of a taste before you add anything.

Now, sit down at the table with no distractions—no screens. Before you take your first bite, again notice the texture, color, and smell of the vegetable, and notice how cooking changes it. Realize that you're about to take a dose of the earth's best medicine and that your body will benefit from just this little bit.

After taking your first bite, put down your fork and give yourself a chance to taste the food. Chew it thoroughly, at least thirty times, before swallowing. As it goes down, pay attention to how you feel when the food gets to your stomach.

As you continue to eat, try to make every bite as mindful as the first. This may take some practice and patience, but it is well worth it.

After you're finished, take a moment to reflect on how your body feels. Are you relaxed? Have you experienced pleasure? Take a minute or two to record your impressions in your notebook.

Explore

To further explore food and your relationship to it, try the following:

- Complete the exercise What Kind of Eater Are You?, available at www.newharbinger.com/47643. This quiz can help you discover how stress and eating are related for you.

- Try the Mindful Snack exercise once a day for a week, then write about it in your notebook.

6

GET INTO YOUR BODY

Movement, especially rhythmic movement, begins long before you're born. In the womb, your heart beat to its own rhythm, independent of your mother's. As soon as you had arms and legs, they were moving—waving, thrusting, swaying in the amniotic fluid day and night. These movements help developing muscles and nerves grow, and make connections in preparation for a lifetime of motion. Long before you made your entry into this world, you spent months learning to move your body and responding to the body's rhythms.

All systems are go during an acute stress response—and, to a lesser degree, in the chronic stress state as well. Keeping your system in a continual state of readiness takes vital resources and energy away from repairing worn-out tissues, fighting infection, growing new cells, digesting and absorbing food, and other life-sustaining activities. So, how do you shift into a more relaxed state and give your body a break? One answer: move it.

The stress response is a true physical state that, in modern society, usually comes from threats you think of, not from immediate threats to your physical safety or well-being. You can cope with these stressors using your mind, but you also need to relieve the physical tension that goes along with chronic stress or it will build and create symptoms like backache, muscle aches and pains, and frequent injuries.

One of the major consequences of chronic stress is insomnia. Regular exercise promotes healthy sleep patterns and can be an effective way to manage insomnia.

What Does Exercise Do?

When I talk about the health benefits of exercise, I mean aerobic exercise, the kind that gets your heart pumping and your blood flowing—things like walking, dancing, running, and bicycling.

Is part of your stress due to concerns about your health? Do you worry about dying of heart disease, cancer, or another chronic, incurable disease? If so, exercise may be part of the solution to your health-related anxieties. If you get moving, you not only get the direct stress-relieving benefits of regular physical activity but you also protect yourself from chronic disease and will probably live a longer, more vital life.

Physical activity stimulates your body to release endorphins, your feel-good neurotransmitters. The benefits continue even when you're not actually exercising: regular physical activity improves mood, even for people with major depression. This is also true for the very old; regular exercise enhances the ability to continue performing the tasks of daily living and promotes positive moods and a sense of meaning in life. Exercise has a strong effect on self-esteem.

Physical fitness seems to function as a type of buffer, or protective factor, between stressful life events and their possible negative impact on physical health. In an early study of people with high blood pressure, Anastasia Georgiades and her colleagues found that people who had exercised regularly for six months fared much better than people who hadn't exercised when confronted with a psychological stressor in the laboratory. The exercisers had lower blood pressure and heart rate before, during, and after the stressor, compared to the nonexercisers.

Setting Exercise Goals

How much exercise do you need? The short answer: probably not as much as you think you do. But really, it depends on your goals. Do you need to lose weight? Do you want to become physically fit at an athletic level? Is there a sport you want to be able to continue well into your older life? Or do you simply want to manage stress and stave off some of the risks of chronic illness?

The first thing to do is decide realistically what you want to gain from regular exercise. Then you have to believe that you will gain these things. Then you have to believe that you can do it.

It's also important to regularly reevaluate your goals, because they may change as your fitness level changes. Many people start with walking for relaxation and better health, get stronger, and then decide they really want to be runners.

One frequent source of confusion about exercise is deciding how hard to work and how often it needs to be done. High-intensity exercise is intimidating to many people. It creates a more dramatic response from the heart and lungs, increases the likelihood of injury, and, in the early phases, it's just not as much fun. It's best to start with moderate-intensity exercise and see where that takes you. If you stay at that level indefinitely, you'll still be reaping excellent benefits to your stress levels and overall health. Furthermore, research suggests that short sessions of exercise are as effective as long sessions for losing weight and increasing physical fitness, as well as for improving mood and sleep, and decreasing stress. In general, the recommendation is strenuous aerobic exercise for thirty to fifty minutes each day. If that's not something you can do now, simple stretching, dancing, or yoga can make a big difference.

Explore

The stress-busting, mood-boosting, sleep-enhancing effects of moving your body are so significant that if you stick with any exercise that you enjoy and can safely perform, you'll benefit. Exercise is for *everyone*, so:

- Use a step tracker to remind you of your movement goal.

- Walk an extra block, take the stairs, dance while you're doing the dishes.

- If you don't know where to start, make an appointment to talk to your doctor about it.

7

EXPRESS YOURSELF

Emotions are natural occurrences that involve body, mind, and spirit. They have a trigger, a beginning, a middle, and an end. Everyone has emotions, but not everyone knows how to express them in a way that serves them. Ideally, feelings lead to self-expression, which develops your self-awareness and boosts your confidence in your ability to weather challenges and losses. Feelings are a source of information and energy you can use to make healthy choices now and in the future.

Your thoughts, feelings, and memories can be a source of stress. Things happen in life that are upsetting, painful, and traumatic. As upsetting things happen, you find ways to manage your feelings about them. Perhaps you, like most people, sometimes do this by setting your emotions aside and not thinking about them very much. It requires a lot of mental effort to not think about things, to store painful memories away and not allow yourself to feel anger, grief, and sadness. It really does cause stress.

Life presents you with challenges and stressors every day, and you respond by coping. As you learned in chapter 2, you can't always control the amount of stress you're exposed to, but you can choose how you cope with it. Some ways of coping are healthier than others.

Socially, emotional suppression creates a mismatch between what's being said and how it's being said. Emotional suppression creates barriers to rapport, intimacy, and the healthy relationships you need in order to thrive. Storing up your feelings and memories of life's upheavals gives them more power. Suppressed feelings and memories become contorted and force themselves into your awareness in ways that are uncomfortable and hard to manage. They can come to you in dreams or obsessive thoughts. An extreme example is post-traumatic stress disorder, a condition marked by the inability to come to terms with traumatic experience, be it a single event or an ongoing situation that exceeds your ability to cope.

It's Normal to Feel

If emotional suppression is not an optimal way to meet the challenges of stress, then what is? What types of coping are best for your physical, emotional, and social health?

There are many ways to express emotion, from the artistic to the verbal. What's important is that you feel what you feel and allow yourself to bring your emotions into the world, where you can acknowledge them and deal with them.

Unless you're severely stressed, it would be unusual for you to be locked into an emotional state for very long. The natural flow of emotions is like waves on a beach. They arrive, sometimes with great power, and then they disperse. Your job is to allow this process to happen organically so that you can make use of the information that feelings carry along with them. You can manage stress much more effectively if you learn to allow your feelings to come and go.

This goes for negative emotions too. Sadness, anger, frustration, resentment: these are all normal emotional states that must be allowed to come and go. Paradoxically, the more you try to deny your negative emotions, the more powerful they become—and the more stress they cause. Many psychological studies have shown that suppression is completely ineffective. A compelling thought or emotion will persist in its demand for attention until it's given its due. Only then will it lose its potency and fade away.

Tracking Negative Emotions

This exercise will help you start to understand your own coping mechanisms and your tolerance for negative emotions. Think of the last time something happened that made you feel angry or frustrated or sad. It needn't be a major trauma, but choose something that made you genuinely upset. The goal is to carefully dissect your reaction to uncover your physical and emotional responses, as well as the story you tell yourself when things go wrong.

Now think about how you thought, felt, and behaved in the moments after the feeling began. As you take the following steps, answer any questions in your notebook.

1. How and where did the emotion reside in your body? Did you feel your muscles get tense, did your heart rate increase, did you need to

pace around, or did you go numb? What did you feel physically? Where in your body did you feel it?

2. Now consider your first impulse in response to your emotion. This is important. Was your first impulse one of escape or approach? That is, did you want to curl up in front of the television with some ice cream, or did you want to call the person and shout it out? How did your mind and thoughts respond to the feelings you were having in your body?

3. Now take a moment to remember how long the feeling lasted. Also, take note of whether you felt a sense of completion when the feeling had passed or whether you still felt vaguely (or acutely) dissatisfied.

4. If you've conjured up the memory in a way that brought on a physical response, take a moment now to relax your body and let the memory go. Take in a long, slow breath, focusing on filling your chest and letting go of any tension there and in your shoulders.

5. Finally, jot some notes about whether the responses you listed in step 2 were helpful. This requires some frank self-awareness and a willingness to look critically at what you say and do. Did you fly off the handle and berate the person you were angry at? Did you smile and say everything was okay even though it wasn't? Part of healthy self-expression is being able to

> notice, name, and discuss emotions
> even when they're uncomfortable.

You can learn effective ways to manage your emotions, but the first thing you need to do is accept your sadness and anger along with your contentment and joy. Sometimes, the best thing you can do is just allow yourself to feel bad for a while and see what lessons there are in the feeling. If the feeling is very strong, it's extremely helpful to engage in strenuous physical activity to release the muscle tension and jitteriness.

Emotional Expression Heals

Self-expression can be difficult, so people often use alcohol or other substances to free themselves to say and do things they ordinarily wouldn't do. Sometimes this is fun and harmless, but it often leads to risky behaviors. Stressful occasions lower your defenses and make it more likely that you'll say or do something hurtful to yourself or others. Bottling up feelings only makes them more concentrated. When they're released, they tend to be harder to control. If self-expression can flow more freely during your everyday life, you'll have less material to release at times of stress or under the influence of alcohol or drugs.

It is important to avoid being abusive with your emotions—to not use their power to manipulate or hurt other people. It's possible to allow yourself to feel anger and grief, and even share these feelings with other people without harming them or the relationship. Some benefits of self-expression include:

Stronger memory: It appears that self-expression frees up your mind from worry and allows you to use the power of working memory for the challenges of daily life.

Meaningful reflection: Self-expression through writing or talking can help you create meaning out of painful events.

Stronger connection to others: Processing problems with other people also strengthens interpersonal bonds. When you are willing and able to express how you feel, you gain many opportunities to get closer to the people in your life.

Improved physical symptoms and immune function: In a landmark study published in the *Journal of the American Medical Association*, Joshua Smyth and his colleagues investigated the possible benefits of writing about stressful events for a group of people with asthma and another group with rheumatoid arthritis.

Patients who wrote about a stressful experience had big changes in every area measured, compared to patients in the control groups.

Disclosing difficult emotions is a key element of many kinds of psychotherapy, including individual therapy, support groups, and art therapy, each of which can be a very effective approach to stress management.

Psychotherapy: In psychotherapy, the therapist and client create a one-on-one relationship grounded in trust and healthy boundaries. Over time, the client feels able to reveal feelings and memories to the therapist in words. Most insurance plans cover at least a few weeks of psychotherapy.

Support groups: Social support is well established as a factor that protects against stress and disease. In support groups, people come together in a controlled environment and talk about themselves. Painful things come up, and they're shared with the group.

Art therapy: Art therapy is a special form of psychotherapy that uses art to express feelings and find solutions to problems. For many people, especially children, this is a good way to get access to feelings that are hard to put into words. Art therapists use drawings, paintings, clay, and other materials to help people express their feelings. Talking about the artwork provides individuals an opportunity to explore issues that they might not otherwise be able to recognize and understand.

Creative Self-Expression

Even without a therapist, you can use the power of disclosure very effectively to manage the stress in your life. You can use focused writing, journaling, and art to express what you're feeling and clarify what you're thinking.

Creative self-expression will eventually strengthen your ability to communicate with other people and be more open in your relationships. It's especially important to be able to express anger and sadness, because these emotions seem to do the most harm if they're denied or suppressed.

You are a creative person simply by virtue of being alive, and you can cultivate your creativity by using your personal experience as raw material. Your thoughts, feelings, perceptions, dreams, ideas, mistakes, and triumphs are rich fodder for growth and worthy of close attention. Here are some ideas to get you started.

Journaling: Making a journal fulfills a need to notice, record, and revisit the events in your life and the world you live in. Disclosure is the key; you bring things out onto paper, where they can be processed, reread, and perhaps eventually destroyed.

Visual journaling: Visual journaling involves the use of drawings, collage, abstract imagery, photographs, and other visual elements in your journal pages. For many people, images enrich the journaling process by adding an emotional element to the page. The benefits of visual journaling are similar to those of art therapy. To get started, simply write different parts of your journal entries in different colored pens. This alone brings the page alive and elicits more emotion. The most important tool for visual journaling is your courage and your spirit. Because you're making art that is only for you, you can freely express yourself and dare yourself to make mistakes.

Storytelling: You can gain perspective on your life by telling personal stories to others. Storytelling can be a special, meaningful activity to share with people you're close to. Here are some ideas for creating a storytelling event. Set aside an evening to gather with your family or a group of your friends for storytelling. Ask everyone to come prepared to share a personal story. Before the storytelling begins, ask that as each person speaks, everyone else listen with their ears, hearts, and minds, with no interruptions. Then, simply take turns telling and hearing stories. Intentional storytelling provides an opportunity for connection, understanding, and self-expression that you simply don't get in everyday life.

Writing About a Stressful Event

This exercise is an effective and easy way to gain mastery over upsets and challenges, and the feelings they bring up. Commit to doing this exercise over the next four days. Resolve to carry this exercise through to its completion and to pay attention to how it affects you by recording your reactions in your notebook.

Here are the steps for each day of writing:

1. Choose a quiet place where you won't be disturbed.

2. Take a moment to choose an experience from your past that was distressing. This will be your target experience, the one you'll write about for the next four days.

Choose something that was upsetting but not so traumatic that you can't think about it without being overwhelmed. Set the intention that you will allow whatever memories, thoughts, and feelings you have about this event to simply flow from you into your writing.

3. Take five minutes or so to sit quietly and relax your body. Don't try to focus on anything; let your gaze be soft and unfocused, or close your eyes.

4. Begin by observing your breath, paying attention to it as you inhale and exhale. You may notice that your shoulders slump slightly, your jaw may slacken, and muscle tension in other areas may loosen. Just allow this to happen.

5. After a few minutes, bring the target experience into your mind. Let yourself remember it as fully as you can, allowing the feelings that go along with the memory to come up. If you start to feel overwhelmed, go back to paying attention to your breath until you feel calmer.

6. Set a timer for twenty minutes. Then, pick up your pen and start to write freely. Don't stop to edit or cross things out—just keep writing. Let your stream of consciousness flow openly onto the paper, even if what you're writing seems to make little sense. This is about the process, not the product. The important thing is to feel free and unencumbered in your expression of what happened and how you felt.

7. Keep writing until the alarm sounds or until you feel a sense of completion.

At first, you may notice that this exercise brings up anxiety or other uncomfortable feelings. As long as they're not severe, see if you can allow these feelings to arise, notice them, and then allow them to pass.

The key to this exercise is to experience bringing an issue to light, allowing it to unfold as a story, being present with the feelings that come along with it, and observing how those feelings have a beginning, a middle, and an end. By doing so, you are practicing active coping and teaching yourself to take a more direct approach to managing stress.

In your journal, you can also write a letter to someone who has caused you pain. This is a private exercise of disclosure: you won't mail the letter. You'll simply give yourself a chance to put your feelings into words as if you were talking to the person, without worrying about the consequences of expressing your feelings, no matter how bitter or petty they may seem to you.

Explore

Accepting that all your emotions are valid is the first step in managing the stress they bring. Consider these questions and write down your responses in your notebook.

- What emotions feel too big or too scary to deal with?

- Which strategies from this chapter will you try to help you feel, tolerate, and safely express your big, scary emotions?

8

CONNECT WITH OTHERS

Relationships can be the best and worst part of human existence, but one thing is certain: their effects are inescapable. We are never free of the influence of others. And this influence is exerted even by the absence of people, as reflected in the health risks of loneliness and isolation. Given the importance of relationships and social connection, it makes sense to learn how they affect stress and health, and to use this understanding to make a better life for yourself and the people you're connected to.

Our human need for connection manifests itself as social support, something that is given from one person to another through some type of relationship, be it professional, intimate, or familial. People give social support consciously, with the intention to be helpful.

There are four major forms of social support:

- *emotional support*, or empathy, love, trust, and caring

- *instrumental support*, or tangible services

- *informational support*, or advice, information, and suggestions

- *appraisal support*, or feedback that helps a person perform self-evaluation

Social Support Heals

There are probably many ways that social support can help you, but two major pathways have been identified. The first is the direct pathway; having good social support improves your mood, your sense of well-being, and the function of your body. The second way is by triggering and fostering better health behaviors; people with good social support tend to take better care of themselves.

Decades of research have shown that social support is probably as important a determinant of how long you live as whether or not you smoke, have high blood pressure, or exercise. Being socially isolated or lonely is very hazardous to your health. People who are lonely tend to have more disease and a shorter life span. There seem to be many reasons for this, some directly physiological and some having to do with decreases in healthy behaviors.

If you're lonely or isolated, it can be very beneficial to seek some form of human contact that feels good to you. If you have social anxiety, counseling could help you. Being part of a support group, a church congregation, or a club can provide enough social support to have positive effects on mood and health. An alternative is to give social support, which can bring feelings of well-being and accomplishment. This is something you can initiate yourself, and it may turn out to be the beginning of new, supportive relationships.

Clearly, social support is important in maintaining your health and managing stress. Let's take a look at how you can build relationships that help you cope with stress rather than causing it.

Sharing Is Caring

Have you ever found that wonderful news just didn't seem real or true until you shared it with someone you loved? And that sharing it truly amplified your joy and excitement about your good fortune? The data show that this act tends to increase your positive mood and your sense of well-being, and it also has benefits for the relationship, including making it more intimate.

So, if your loved one shares good news with you, be sure to communicate your genuine happiness. If you don't feel happy about your partner's good news, this may signal real problems in the relationship. Similarly, if your good news is frequently met by neutral, disinterested, or outright negative responses by your partner, there may be a real need to explore issues of intimacy, competitiveness, envy, and other possible problems in the relationship. In the long run, a lack of support for your good fortune can be almost as harmful to you and your relationship as a lack of support when things go wrong.

Ask for What You Want

Here's an exercise to help you identify your social support preferences and needs. You'll need your notebook for this exercise. Begin by remembering a stressful incident that occurred in the last week or two. Choose an event that, afterward, you told someone about. It doesn't have to be a dramatic event, just something that bothered you. Now, write a paragraph about the incident.

After you're done, take a minute to reread what you just wrote, and answer the following questions:

1. Did you write a dry narrative based on the facts?

2. Did you write about how you felt as the event was happening?

3. Did you write about blame or responsibility for the event, ascribing it either to yourself or to someone or something outside of yourself?

4. Did you include a lot of sensory detail in your story?

Now, think about the person you told the story to. Describe your relationship with this person in a sentence or two. Now, thinking back, how did you tell the story to this person? Answer the same four questions about that conversation. Finally, note the response you got from the person with whom you shared the story.

By analyzing what you've written, you can get some insight into your style of social support seeking and whether your needs are being met. Looking at the first set of questions, notice whether you described the event in emotional or factual terms. Focusing on blame or responsibility may trigger a greater need for practical processing of the event. If you had a lot of sensory detail in your story, the event may have been a traumatic experience that you need to process emotionally to better organize and store the memory to make it less disturbing.

Now, look at the way you told the story to the other person. Was it in the same style as your written story? If not, you may be changing your delivery in an attempt to match what you perceive as the other person's style of coping with stress. This may be helpful in getting your point across, but it may not elicit the type of support *you* need. If you're feeling upset but you need to tell your story in dry, factual terms to get the other person to listen to you, you may be missing out on the emotional validation and comfort you're looking for.

Look at your analysis of the other person's response. This will give you more information about the degree of compatibility you have with your confidante. If you were looking for emotional succor and the person asked for factual information and gave advice, you may have been frustrated and disappointed by the encounter. Consider the idea that often people give you what they think will be helpful, based on what helps them.

Explore

Using the information from this chapter, reflect:

- What helps you most when you're stressed (advice, a hug, just talking it out, some personal space, etc.)? Who in your life could give this help to you?

- How might you ask particular people for what you need?

- Now give asking for help a try: choose three small to medium requests, plan who and how you'll ask, and then go for it. Later, write about how it went and how you might practice asking for what you need the next time.

9

TRAIN YOUR BRAIN

As you learned in the introduction, the acute stress response is highly adaptive and lifesaving, but expensive in terms of the resources your body needs to heal, grow, regenerate, and nourish itself. Animals in their natural environments move in and out of these acute stress reactions naturally, but we humans, with our ability to ruminate and fret over our problems, often get locked into a stress response that goes on and on. *Mind-body techniques* can free us from that stuck-in-stress response.

Most mind-body techniques have the same goal: to shift you from an activated, stressed state to a calm, relaxed one. This helps in at least two ways: First, the techniques give you a stress break while you are doing them. Second, regular practice leads to less nervous system activation the rest of the day, counteracting the harmful health effects of stress and hassles.

Here are four mind-body techniques you can use every day.

The relaxation response: This technique is easy to learn and do. To invite relaxation, first focus your awareness on a phrase, a sound, or a word. Second, stay with your focus—even when thoughts arise. Gently dismiss any intruding thoughts and return to your word, phrase, or sound. That's it. It's best to practice for ten to twenty minutes a day—and regular practice is key to making this automatic.

Breath work: Breathing happens at the boundary between your autonomic (involuntary) nervous system and your voluntary, or conscious, actions. You can decide *how* to breathe, but you don't stop breathing when you stop thinking about it. It's easy to learn how to make your breathing deeper, slower, and more regular, and this kind of breathing leads to pronounced relaxation that you can feel in your whole body even as it calms and steadies your mind. Again, practicing any kind of breath work for just minutes a day when you're not especially stressed—and using it in moments of stress—can noticeably reduce your stress overall.

Guided imagery: Doing guided imagery is like watching a movie in your mind. And your body will respond to the content of the imagery in turn. Guided imagery can be *passive*, such as when you listen to a recorded or live script, or *active*, such as when you choose a situation and imagine it happening. Imagery work can produce powerful physiological changes, including strong influences on immune function. It can also help you gain insight into stressful situations and physical problems. Guided imagery apps and videos are plentiful on the web—try a few that look good to you, and choose one or two to add to a daily or weekly practice.

Autogenic training: Autogenic training is a form of self-hypnosis in which you train your nervous system to calm down whenever you want it to. It's a reliable, powerful tool for relaxation that many people really enjoy. The idea is that you practice the technique in a safe, relaxed environment for a few weeks. Once you're comfortable with it, you can start using it in your daily life.

Practice autogenic training at home first, learning simple commands and associating them with imagery to make the commands more integrated with your brain's way of communicating. You'll find that you're able to get relaxed easily using the commands after a few weeks, and then you can take it on the road. To start, try the following exercise, practicing this technique every day, at the same time of day.

Autogenic Training

Sit in a comfortable chair. I don't recommend lying down, because it's best not to fall asleep while you're learning the technique. Later, however, you can use it to help yourself get to sleep if you have insomnia.

Begin by closing your eyes and focusing on your body and how it feels. Briefly run from head to toes, noting whether you need to loosen your clothes or adjust your position so your muscles can relax. Once you're comfortable, shift your attention to your breathing. Pay attention to the air coming into your lungs, filling your chest, and slowly moving out of your body, carrying away things you don't need. Think about your breath getting a little slower and deeper, but don't force it to change.

If thoughts come into your head (and they will), tell yourself you'll deal with them later. Just say, *Not now*, and let the thoughts wander off.

Now, repeat each of the following phrases to yourself three times. While you're repeating the phrases, create an image in your mind of the thing happening. For example, for "My hands are soft and warm," you might imagine them cupped around a bowl of soup. Use more than one sense. What does it look like? How does it smell? At first, it may be hard to remember the phrases, so you will have to pause to look at this book, but it won't be long before you have them memorized. Remember, say each one three times to yourself before moving on to the next one.

> *My hands are soft and warm... I am at peace.*
>
> *My legs are heavy and warm... I am at peace.*
>
> *My breathing is deep and calm... I am at peace.*

My forehead is cool... I am at peace.

My belly is soft and warm... I am at peace.

My body is always healing itself... I am at peace.

Before you open your eyes and come back to your regular state of awareness, take a minute to scan your body again and notice how it feels to be deeply relaxed. The more familiar you get with this feeling, the easier it will be for you to recognize when you need to create it.

After you've practiced daily for a couple of weeks, try using autogenic training out in the world in situations that normally cause you stress. The easiest way to do this is to choose the phrase you like best and make it a sort of mantra. I personally like "I am at peace" or "I am peace." When I'm in traffic or another stressful situation, I interrupt my busy mind and focus on my hands. I think about them getting warm, and I say to myself, *I am at peace.* In moments, my hands get warmer and I feel calmer.

Explore

Experiment with the four mind-body training techniques in this chapter, and write about your experiences. Does one seem to work better than the others to lower your overall stress? Choose one to practice daily for at least the next month, so that it's there for you when you need it most.

10

RISE ABOVE

Stressful events are all around you all the time, yet many people seem to be able to put them in perspective and continue growing, thriving, and being happy, even in the worst of circumstances. How do they do it? Thriving is served, for many people, by a sense of wonder, inspiration, awe, and connection with a greater aspect of reality than what is immediately obvious. These things add up to spirituality and often are acted out as religion. You can integrate these benefits into your life regardless of your particular beliefs.

Transcendence may be the key to developing a spiritual orientation to life. Transcendent experience has been defined many ways, but it often includes the extension of the boundaries of the self beyond the physical body, either to vast spaces within or through connection with infinite space beyond the individual. The experience is rarely frightening and usually brings with it a sense of profound connection and well-being.

There has been an explosion of interest in the ways that spirituality and religion can improve health and long-term well-being. Research suggests that religious and spiritual experience can have both physiological and psychological benefits. How can this be?

Mind, Body ... and Spirit

People who engage in religious and spiritual activities experience benefits to many body systems, including the cardiovascular, nervous, endocrine, and immune systems. Nobody is sure exactly how religious activity, spirituality, and physiological function are connected. Perhaps going to church is a relaxing experience similar to a session of meditation, with long-lasting physical effects. Perhaps being spiritually oriented contributes to better mood states; we know that positive mood states tend to protect against stress-related physical changes. Religion and spirituality have psychological benefits as well as.

So, what's the active ingredient in religiousness and spirituality that is responsible for these positive effects? Most likely, it is a heightened sense of meaning and coherence in the world. *Meaning-based coping* is recognized as a highly adaptive strategy that can lead to better moods and healthier behaviors. It may be that viewing life as a coherent, meaningful enterprise gives people a stronger sense of purpose, because their intentions and beliefs guide behaviors and provide a rationale for the choices they make.

There are many definitions of spirituality, but they all seem to include some sense of a reality that transcends everyday experience. When life's stresses and problems are put in a bigger perspective—eternity, ultimate truth, ultimate goodness, heaven and hell—they seem smaller and, for many people, somehow more manageable.

What does this mean for you? Perhaps, you might want to cultivate a sense of spiritual connection and meaning in your life. There are many ways to do that, from reading books about spirituality to finding a community to join, to taking a yoga class, to joining a church. It's up to you, but if you feel drawn to it, you will be able to find some way to nurture your spiritual longing.

Enhancing Your Spirituality

Prayer is a form of spiritual practice that doesn't have to be aligned with any particular religion, although it is a mainstay of pretty much every religion on earth. More important than the type of prayer is how it feels when you're doing it. If it leads to a greater sense of connection and meaning, it's probably having a beneficial effect.

Prayer is something you can do anytime, anywhere. All you need to do is sit quietly and allow your mind to slow down. Decide ahead of time what kind of prayer you want to do. Many of the people I've worked with start with prayers of thanksgiving. I think this is a beautiful way to start a prayer practice. It can be as simple as bowing your head briefly before you eat. Expressing gratitude is a great way to remind yourself that your life is a miracle and that, no matter what's going on, things could be worse.

Being spiritual, adopting a religious practice, being a stressed-out maniac—these are all choices we make from moment to moment. It's up to you to exert whatever control you can to make your life as peaceful, generous, and happy as it can be.

Explore

To assess your sense of spiritual meaning, visit www.newharbinger.com/47643 to download the exercise Does Life Have Meaning? After you have completed the questionnaire, consider these questions:

- What have you done in the past to strengthen your spiritual well-being?

- What do you do now?

- How do you think a strong sense of spiritual meaning would help you live your best life?

STRESS TOOL KIT

On the lines on the next couple of pages, name the stress management tips you've learned that work best for you (include the page number in this book so you can remind yourself easily). Put a checkmark next to the ones that give you quick relief and a star next to the ones that seem to keep you calm when you do them regularly.

_____

_____

_____

_____

_____

_____

Stress Tool Kit

Claire Michaels Wheeler, MD, PhD, is an instructor at Oregon Health and Science University School of Medicine, and Portland State University; as well as a faculty member at The Center for MindBody Medicine in Washington, DC.

Real change *is* possible

For more than forty-five years, New Harbinger has published proven-effective self-help books and pioneering workbooks to help readers of all ages and backgrounds improve mental health and well-being, and achieve lasting personal growth. In addition, our spirituality books offer profound guidance for deepening awareness and cultivating healing, self-discovery, and fulfillment.

Founded by psychologist Matthew McKay and Patrick Fanning, New Harbinger is proud to be an independent, employee-owned company. Our books reflect our core values of integrity, innovation, commitment, sustainability, compassion, and trust. Written by leaders in the field and recommended by therapists worldwide, New Harbinger books are practical, accessible, and provide real tools for real change.

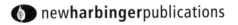